BLOOD SUGAR DIET SOLUTION FOR WOMEN

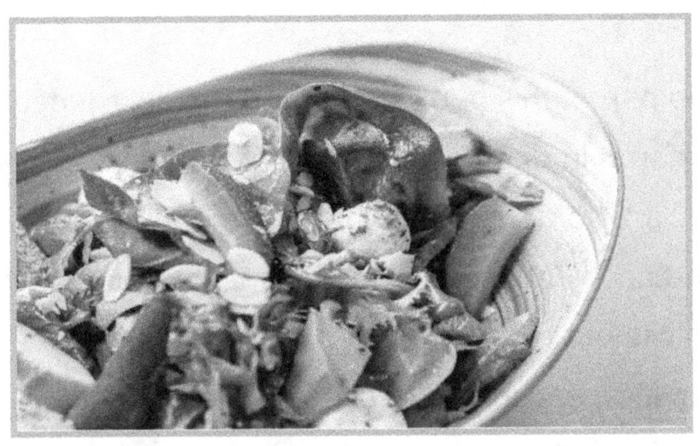

A 14-Day Meal Plan Journey in
Taking Control and
Transforming your Health

Karla Mayer

TABLE OF CONTENT

INTRODUCTION

The book "Blood Sugar Diet Solution for Women" is a comprehensive guide focused on revitalizing women's health and reclaiming their bodies by balancing blood sugar levels. It offers a female-centered approach to managing blood sugar levels and improving overall health through diet, lifestyle, and personalized strategies. The book provides advice on diet, green living, supplements, medication, exercise, stress-reducing strategies, a menu plan, recipes, and a 14 days action plan. The book presents an ultra-healthy program for losing weight, preventing disease, and feeling great, with a specific focus on women's health. It is designed to help women take control of their blood sugar and lead a healthy lifestyle.

This guide is not just a manual but a beacon of empowerment for women seeking to reclaim control over their health destinies. We delve into the science behind blood sugar regulation, unraveling the impact on energy levels, mood swings, and overall vitality. More than a mere diet plan, this book introduces a lifestyle solution—a comprehensive approach that embraces nourishment for the body, mind, and soul.

As we turn the pages, let us embark on a journey that goes beyond mere dietary restrictions, inviting women to embrace a sustainable, empowering, and fulfilling path to well-being. Together, let's unlock the secrets to stable blood sugar and embrace a life where vitality and resilience become the guiding stars on our health voyage.

CHAPTER ONE

Understanding Blood Sugar

Blood sugar in women encompasses various aspects related to blood sugar levels, their impact on women's health, and strategies for managing them. Blood sugar, or glucose, is a vital source of energy for the body's cells and is regulated by insulin, a hormone produced by the pancreas. In women, several factors can influence blood sugar levels, including hormonal changes, pregnancy, menopause, and polycystic ovary syndrome (PCOS).

Maintaining healthy blood sugar levels is crucial for women's overall well-being, as imbalances can lead to various health issues, including gestational diabetes, type 2 diabetes, heart disease, and PCOS. Therefore, a balanced blood sugar diet solution for women typically involves a combination of healthy eating, regular physical activity, stress management, adequate sleep, and, in some cases, medication or insulin therapy.

In women, as in men, blood sugar levels are influenced by factors such as diet, physical activity, and overall health.

Here are key points regarding blood sugar in women:

Normal Blood Sugar Levels:

Fasting Blood Sugar: Typically, normal fasting blood sugar levels range from 70 to 100 milligrams per deciliter (mg/dL).

Postprandial (After Eating): Blood sugar levels may rise temporarily after meals, but they should return to fasting levels within a few hours.

Hormonal Influence:

Blood sugar regulation is greatly aided by hormones like glucagon and insulin. Insulin helps cells absorb glucose from the bloodstream, while glucagon raises blood sugar levels when needed.

Hormonal fluctuations during the menstrual cycle can affect insulin sensitivity, potentially leading to variations in blood sugar levels.

Pregnancy and Gestational Diabetes:

During pregnancy, hormonal changes can impact insulin sensitivity, and women may develop gestational diabetes. This condition requires careful monitoring of blood sugar levels to avoid complications for both the mother and the baby.

Polycystic Ovary Syndrome (PCOS):

PCOS is a common hormonal disorder in women that can be associated with insulin resistance, leading to elevated blood sugar levels. Proper management includes lifestyle changes and, in some cases, medication.

Menopause and Diabetes Risk:

Menopausal changes can affect insulin sensitivity, potentially increasing the risk of developing diabetes. Regular health check-ups and a healthy lifestyle become crucial during this phase.

Symptoms of High/Low Blood Sugar:

Hyperglycemia, or high blood sugar, can cause symptoms like excessive thirst, frequent urination, exhaustion, and impaired vision.

Low Blood Sugar (Hypoglycemia): Symptoms may include shakiness, sweating, irritability, and confusion.

Management and Prevention:

Lifestyle factors such as a balanced diet, regular physical activity, and maintaining a healthy weight are key components of blood sugar management and prevention of diabetes.

Regular Monitoring:

For individuals with diabetes or at risk, regular monitoring of blood sugar levels is essential to manage the condition effectively.

CHAPTER TWO

The Role of Nutrition in Regulating Blood Sugar Control

The role of nutrition in regulating blood sugar is crucial for overall health, especially for individuals who have conditions like diabetes or those at risk of developing it. Blood sugar, or glucose, is the primary source of energy for our body's cells, and maintaining stable blood sugar levels is essential for proper functioning. Here's an in-depth look at the key aspects of how nutrition influences blood sugar regulation:

Carbohydrates:
Carbohydrates are the main macronutrient that significantly impacts blood sugar levels. They are broken down into glucose during digestion. Simple carbohydrates (sugars) cause a rapid spike in blood sugar, while complex carbohydrates (found in whole grains, fruits,

and vegetables) provide a slower, more sustained release of glucose.

Fiber:

Dietary fiber, found in fruits, vegetables, whole grains, and legumes, slows down the digestion and absorption of carbohydrates.
This helps prevent rapid spikes in blood sugar and promotes better blood sugar control.

Protein:

Including protein in meals can help stabilize blood sugar levels by slowing down the absorption of carbohydrates.
Protein-rich foods, such as lean meats, fish, eggs, and plant-based sources like beans and tofu, are important components of a balanced diet.

Fats:

Healthy fats, such as those found in avocados, nuts, seeds, and olive oil, can contribute to blood sugar stability.

Fats slow down the digestion of food, preventing quick spikes in blood sugar levels.

Meal Timing and Portion Control:

Eating regular, balanced meals throughout the day helps regulate blood sugar. Skipping meals or consuming large portions can lead to erratic blood sugar levels.

Portion control is essential, as overeating can overwhelm the body's ability to manage blood sugar effectively.

Glycemic Index (GI):

The glycemic index calculates the rate at which a specific food elevates blood sugar. Foods with a high GI cause a rapid spike, while those with a low GI release glucose more slowly.

Choosing low-GI foods, such as whole grains, legumes, and non-starchy vegetables, can contribute to better blood sugar control.

Hydration:

Staying well-hydrated supports overall health and can help regulate blood sugar levels. Water is the best choice, while sugary drinks should be limited.

Individualized Nutrition Plans:

The ideal nutrition plan for blood sugar regulation can vary among individuals. Factors such as age, weight, physical activity, and any existing health conditions should be considered when creating a personalized approach.

Monitoring and Adaptation:

Regular monitoring of blood sugar levels is crucial for individuals with diabetes. This allows for adjustments to nutrition plans, medication, or lifestyle to maintain optimal control.

In summary, a well-balanced diet with a focus on whole, nutrient-dense foods, combined with proper meal timing and portion control, plays a central role in regulating blood sugar levels. Individualized nutrition plans, in consultation with healthcare professionals, are key for effectively managing blood sugar and promoting overall health.

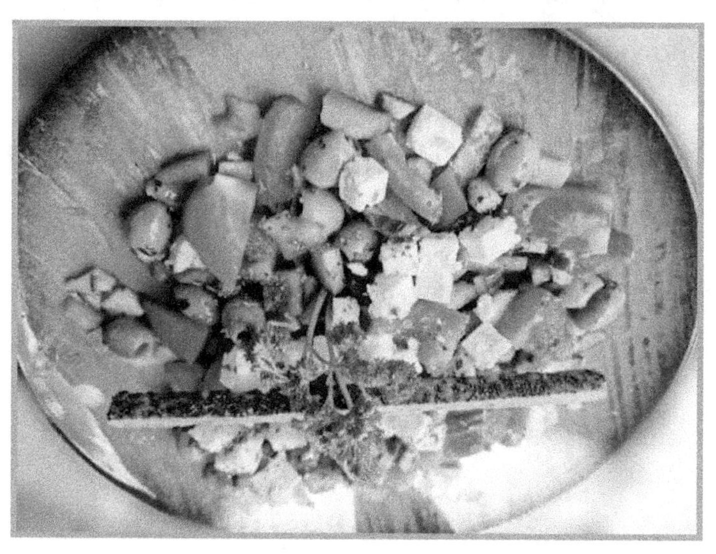

CHAPTER THREE

Low Carb in Blood Sugar Control

Low-carb diets have been shown to be effective in controlling blood sugar levels in people with diabetes, including women. Compared to other foods, carbohydrates cause blood glucose to rise more, requiring the body to create more insulin in order to digest them. Reducing carb intake can help stabilize blood glucose and counteract some other effects of diabetes, such as weight gain and heart disease.

A low-carb diet for diabetes can effectively help manage type 1 and type 2 diabetes by improving blood sugar management.

It has been demonstrated that increasing daily carbohydrate consumption of 20–90 grams helps improve blood sugar control in diabetics. However, it is best to test and adjust the carb intake based on personal tolerance. A healthy low-carb diet should include nutrient-dense, high-fiber carb sources, like vegetables, berries, nuts, and seeds

In a trial of two low-carb diets, both the keto and Mediterranean diets were similarly effective in controlling blood glucose. The stricter carbohydrate limitations of Keto did not yield any significant health advantages overall.

It is important to note that low-carb diets may cause some people to feel hungry, moody, or have trouble concentrating. Anyone who wants to try a low-carb diet to help manage diabetes may want to speak to a doctor or healthcare professional to ensure they get all the nutrients they need.

Here are some key points to consider regarding low-carb diets and blood sugar control:

Reduced Carbohydrate Intake:
Low-carb diets typically limit the intake of carbohydrates, which are broken down into glucose in the body. By reducing carb intake,

there is less glucose produced, leading to lower blood sugar levels.

Improved Insulin Sensitivity:
Carbohydrates have a direct impact on insulin levels. A low-carb diet can improve insulin sensitivity, helping the body use insulin more effectively to regulate blood sugar.

Stable Blood Sugar Levels:
Low-carb diets can result in more stable blood sugar levels throughout the day, reducing the likelihood of spikes and crashes.Those who have diabetes would especially benefit from this.

Weight Management:
Diets low in carbohydrates can help with weight loss or maintenance. Excess body weight is often linked to insulin resistance, and losing weight can improve the body's response to insulin.

Reduction in Medication:

Some individuals on low-carb diets may find that they require less medication to control their blood sugar. It's crucial to work closely with healthcare professionals to adjust medication as needed.

Focus on Healthy Fats and Proteins:

While low-carb diets restrict carbohydrates, they often emphasize healthy fats and proteins. This can help maintain energy levels and provide essential nutrients while avoiding blood sugar spikes.

Types of Low-Carb Diets:

There are various low-carb diets, such as the ketogenic diet (very low-carb, high-fat), Atkins, and low-glycemic index diets. Each has its own approach to carbohydrate restriction.

Individual Variability:

It's important to note that individual responses to low-carb diets can vary. Some people may experience significant benefits, while others may not respond as well. A person's lifestyle, general health, and heredity are all important factors.

Consultation with Healthcare Professionals:

Before making significant changes to your diet, especially if you have diabetes or other health conditions, it's essential to consult with healthcare professionals. They are able to offer tailored guidance according to your particular medical requirements.

It's crucial to recognize that a low-carb diet may not be suitable for everyone, and the goal should be to find a sustainable and balanced approach to blood sugar control that aligns with individual health needs and preferences.Healthcare professionals should

always be consulted before making major
dietary adjustments.

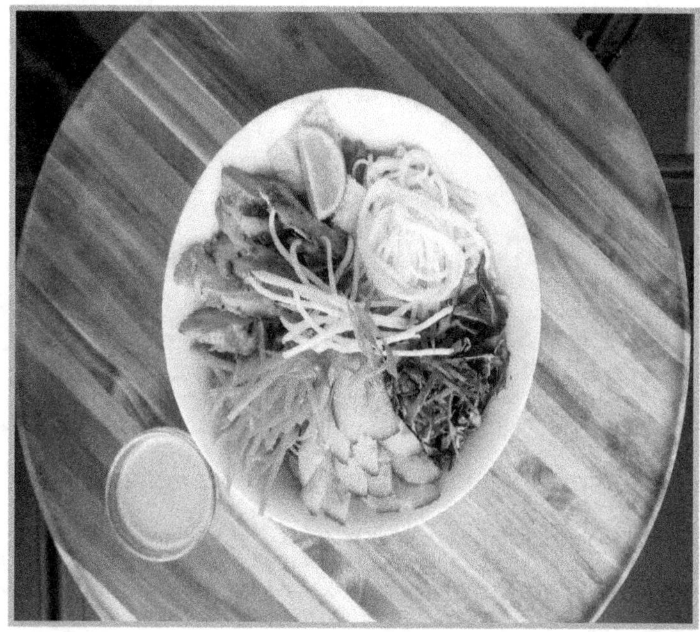

CHAPTER FOUR

Exercise and Its Impact on Blood Sugar Control

Exercise plays a crucial role in blood sugar control for both men and women, but there are certain considerations and effects that may be particularly relevant for women. Here are some key points to consider:

Insulin Sensitivity:

Regular physical activity improves insulin sensitivity, allowing cells to more effectively use glucose for energy. This is essential for blood sugar control.

Women who engage in regular exercise may experience enhanced insulin sensitivity, which can help in managing blood sugar levels more effectively.

Hormonal Influences:

Women's hormonal fluctuations, especially during the menstrual cycle, can impact blood sugar levels and insulin sensitivity.

Regular exercise can help mitigate these hormonal effects and contribute to more stable blood sugar levels.

Weight Management:

Sustaining a healthy weight is crucial for managing blood sugar levels. . Exercise helps with weight management by burning calories and promoting lean muscle mass.

Women may face unique challenges related to weight management, and exercise can be an effective tool in addressing these challenges.

Cardiovascular Health:

Exercise improves cardiovascular health, reducing the risk of heart disease and related complications, which are often associated with diabetes.

Cardiovascular exercise, such as walking, running, or cycling, can be particularly beneficial for women in promoting heart health.

Type of Exercise:
Both aerobic (cardio) and resistance training exercises have positive effects on blood sugar control.
Resistance training, in particular, helps build muscle, which can contribute to improved glucose metabolism.
Women should include a combination of aerobic and resistance exercises in their routine for overall health benefits.

Post-Exercise Blood Sugar Levels:
In some cases, intense or prolonged exercise might cause temporary increases in blood sugar levels due to the release of stress hormones. However, regular exercise generally leads to better long-term blood sugar control.

It's essential for women with diabetes or those at risk to monitor their blood sugar levels closely, especially after new or intense exercise routines.

Consistency is Key:

Consistent, moderate-intensity exercise is often more sustainable and can lead to better long-term blood sugar control.

Finding activities that women enjoy and can incorporate into their lifestyle is crucial for adherence to an exercise routine.

Consultation with Healthcare Professionals:

Women with pre-existing health conditions or those who are pregnant should consult with their healthcare providers before starting a new exercise regimen.

In summary, exercise is a powerful tool for blood sugar control in women. Combining regular physical activity with a balanced diet and overall healthy lifestyle choices can contribute to better glucose metabolism and overall well-being. Individual considerations and health status should always be taken into account when designing an exercise plan, and consulting with healthcare professionals is advisable.

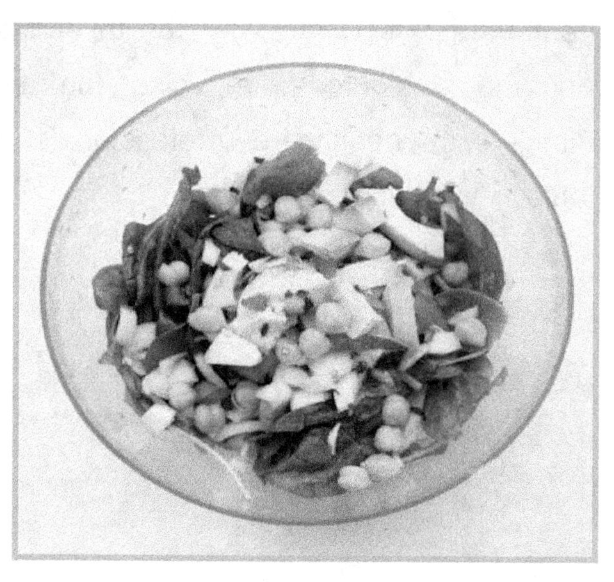

CHAPTER FIVE

Weight Management in Blood Sugar Control

Weight management is particularly important for women in the context of blood sugar control, especially considering factors such as hormonal fluctuations, pregnancy, and the increased risk of developing gestational diabetes or type 2 diabetes. For women specifically, take into account the following:

Hormonal Influences:

Hormonal changes, such as those associated with the menstrual cycle, pregnancy, and menopause, can impact insulin sensitivity and blood sugar levels. Women may experience changes in appetite and metabolism during different phases of their menstrual cycle, emphasizing the importance of consistent weight management strategies.

Gestational Diabetes:

Pregnancy increases insulin resistance, and some women may develop gestational diabetes, a temporary form of diabetes that occurs during pregnancy. Maintaining a healthy weight before and during pregnancy is crucial for preventing gestational diabetes and managing blood sugar levels during this critical period.

Postpartum Weight Management:

After childbirth, women may face challenges related to postpartum weight retention. Addressing postpartum weight management is important not only for general health but also for reducing the risk of developing type 2 diabetes in the future.

Polycystic Ovary Syndrome (PCOS):

PCOS is a common hormonal disorder among women of reproductive age that is associated with insulin resistance. Weight management is often a key component in managing PCOS and improving insulin sensitivity. Lifestyle modifications, including weight loss, regular exercise, and a balanced diet, can be beneficial for women with PCOS.

Age-Related Changes:
As women age, there may be changes in metabolism and body composition. Maintaining a healthy weight and engaging in regular physical activity can help counteract age-related changes and support optimal blood sugar control.

Nutrition and Dietary Choices:
Women should pay attention to their nutritional needs, especially during different life stages. A balanced diet that includes whole grains, lean proteins, healthy fats, and a variety of fruits and vegetables can contribute to weight management and blood sugar control.

Individualized Approaches:

Women may benefit from individualized approaches to weight management based on their unique health circumstances, including any existing medical conditions, medications, and reproductive health concerns. Consulting with healthcare professionals, such as registered dietitians or endocrinologists, can help tailor strategies to individual needs.

Regular Physical Activity:

Physical activity is crucial for both weight management and blood sugar control. Engaging in regular exercise can enhance insulin sensitivity, help with weight loss or maintenance, and contribute to overall well-being.

It's important for women to approach weight management in the context of blood sugar control as part of a holistic and personalized lifestyle plan. Consulting with healthcare professionals, including gynecologists, endocrinologists, and registered dietitians, can provide tailored guidance to support women in achieving and maintaining a healthy weight and optimal blood sugar levels throughout their life stages.

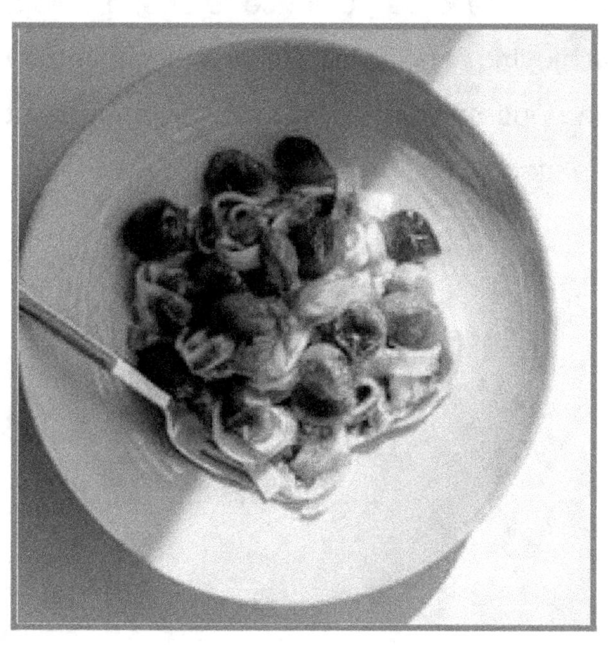

CHAPTER SIX

Intermittent Fasting in Blood Sugar Solution

An eating pattern known as intermittent fasting (IF) alternates between times when one eats and when one fasts. It has gained popularity for its potential benefits in various aspects of health, including blood sugar management. However, it's crucial to note that individual responses to intermittent fasting can vary, and consulting with a healthcare professional is important, especially for women with blood sugar concerns.

Here are some aspects of intermittent fasting in the context of blood sugar management:

Insulin Sensitivity:

Intermittent fasting may help improve insulin sensitivity, which is essential for managing blood sugar levels. By giving the body a break from constant food intake, IF can potentially reduce insulin resistance, allowing cells to better respond to insulin and regulate blood sugar more effectively.

Reduced Blood Sugar Spikes:
IF may contribute to more stable blood sugar levels by preventing frequent spikes that occur with regular meals throughout the day. By restricting the eating window, there is less opportunity for excessive carbohydrate consumption, which can contribute to elevated blood sugar levels.

Weight Management:
Sustaining a healthy weight is essential for managing blood sugar levels. Intermittent fasting may help some individuals achieve weight loss or weight maintenance by regulating calorie intake and promoting fat utilization for energy. Higher blood sugar levels

and insulin resistance can be linked to excess body weight.

Inflammation Reduction:
Chronic inflammation is linked to insulin resistance and other metabolic issues. Some studies suggest that intermittent fasting may help reduce inflammation in the body, potentially benefiting those with blood sugar concerns.

Hormonal Balance:
Hormones play a significant role in blood sugar regulation. Intermittent fasting can impact hormonal balance, potentially improving insulin and leptin sensitivity. Leptin is a hormone that helps regulate appetite and energy balance.

Cautions for Women:
Women may experience hormonal fluctuations that can be influenced by fasting. Some women may find that certain fasting protocols,

such as daily intermittent fasting, may not be suitable for them, especially if they have irregular menstrual cycles or hormonal imbalances. It's essential for women to listen to their bodies and consult healthcare professionals to ensure that intermittent fasting is appropriate for their individual circumstances.

Personalization and Monitoring:
Intermittent fasting is not a one-size-fits-all approach. The effectiveness of IF can vary from person to person. Regular monitoring of blood sugar levels, along with professional guidance, is crucial to ensure that the chosen fasting pattern aligns with individual health needs.

In summary, while intermittent fasting may offer potential benefits for blood sugar management, it's essential for women to approach it cautiously and consider individual health factors. Consulting with a healthcare provider or a registered dietitian can help create a personalized approach to intermittent fasting that addresses specific concerns and ensures overall well-being.

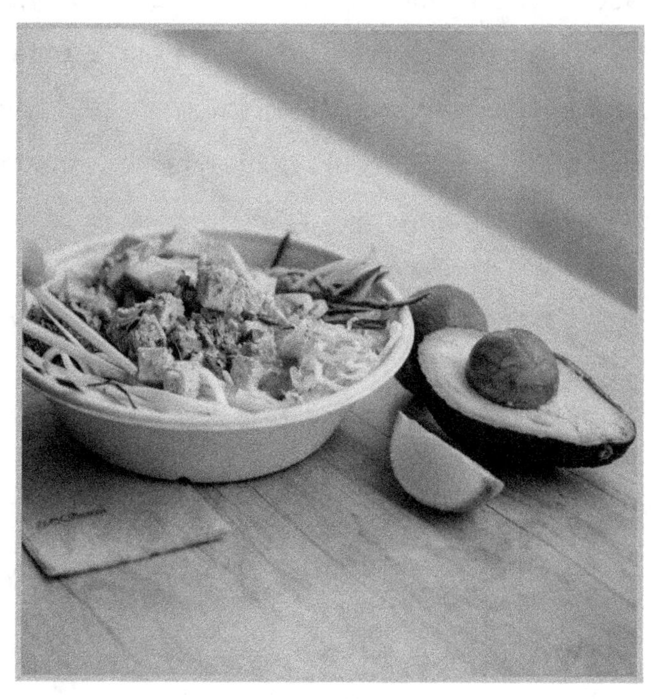

CHAPTER SEVEN

Natural Products and Supplements for Blood Sugar Control

Controlling blood sugar levels is essential for good health in general, especially for those who already have diabetes or are at risk of getting it. Natural products and supplements are often explored as complementary approaches to help control blood sugar levels. It's essential to note that while some of these supplements may show promising results in studies, they should not replace conventional medical treatments, and individuals should consult with their healthcare provider before incorporating them into their routine.

Cinnamon:

Studies suggest that cinnamon may help improve insulin sensitivity and lower blood sugar levels.

It can be sprinkled on food or taken as a supplement, but the dosage should be monitored to avoid potential side effects.

Chromium:

A tiny element called chromium affects how well insulin works.

Some studies indicate that chromium supplementation may help improve insulin sensitivity, but more research is needed.

Alpha-Lipoic Acid (ALA):

ALA is an antioxidant that may help improve insulin sensitivity and reduce inflammation.

It is found in certain foods like spinach and broccoli, and supplements are also available.

Berberine:

Berberine is a compound found in several plants and has been studied for its potential to lower blood sugar levels.

It may work similarly to some pharmaceutical medications used for diabetes.

Fenugreek:

Soluble fiber included in fenugreek seeds has the potential to reduce blood sugar levels.

Some studies suggest that fenugreek supplements may be beneficial for people with diabetes.

Bitter Melon:

Bitter melon is a fruit that has been traditionally used in some cultures for its potential anti-diabetic properties.

Further research is necessary, but it might help reduce blood sugar levels.

Magnesium:

Magnesium is an essential mineral involved in various bodily functions, including glucose metabolism.

Some studies suggest that magnesium supplementation may have a modest effect on blood sugar control.

Vitamin D:

Insulin resistance has been linked to vitamin D insufficiency.

Sun exposure and dietary sources are natural ways to get vitamin D, but supplements may be necessary for some individuals.

Ginseng:

Certain types of ginseng, such as American ginseng and Korean ginseng, have been studied for their potential to improve insulin sensitivity.

Probiotics:

Some research suggests that the balance of gut bacteria may influence blood sugar levels. Probiotics, found in fermented foods or supplements, may positively impact gut health.

It's crucial to approach these supplements with caution, as individual responses can vary, and interactions with medications may occur. It is advisable to speak with a healthcare provider before beginning any new supplement regimen. Additionally, lifestyle factors such as a balanced diet, regular physical activity, and maintaining a healthy weight are fundamental components of blood sugar control.

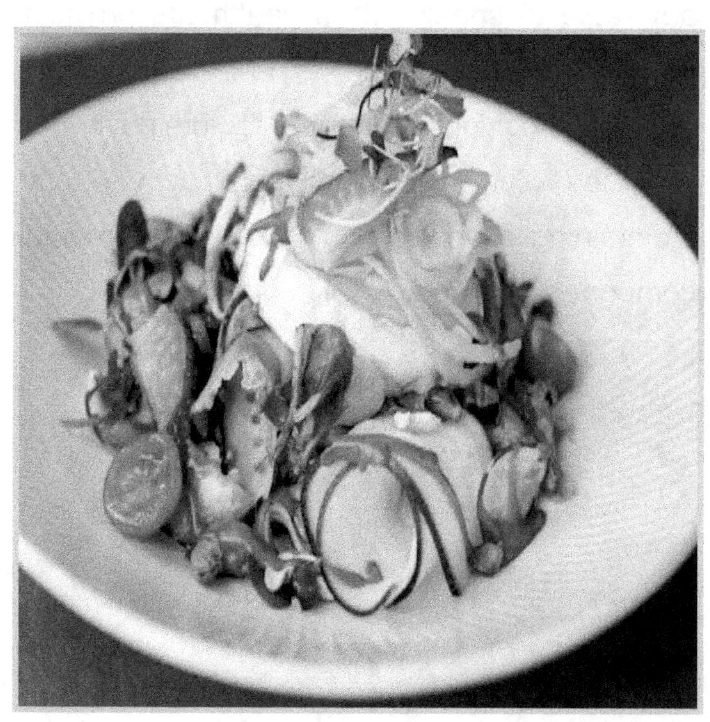

CHAPTER EIGHT

Adapting the Blood Sugar Diet to Women's Specific Needs

Adapting the Blood Sugar Diet to women's specific needs involves recognizing the unique hormonal and physiological aspects of women that can impact blood sugar levels and overall health. The Blood Sugar Diet, which focuses on managing blood sugar through dietary changes, can be tailored to better suit women's requirements for optimal well-being. Adapting the Blood Sugar Diet to women's specific needs involves recognizing and accommodating the unique aspects of women's health. Customizing the diet based on hormonal fluctuations, nutritional needs, and individual requirements can contribute to better blood sugar control and overall well-being.

Here are some considerations and tips for adapting the Blood Sugar Diet for women:

1. Understanding Hormonal Changes:

Hormonal changes occur in women during the menstrual cycle, pregnancy, and menopause.These changes can influence insulin sensitivity and blood sugar levels. Adjust the diet based on these hormonal shifts, emphasizing nutrient-dense foods during vulnerable times, such as increasing complex carbohydrates during the menstrual phase to address cravings.

2. Balancing Macronutrients:

Make sure your consumption of the macronutrients—fats, proteins, and carbohydrates—is well-balanced. While the Blood Sugar Diet typically encourages a low-carbohydrate approach, it's essential to consider individual needs. Some women may benefit from slightly higher carbohydrate intake, especially those with intense physical activity or during specific phases of the menstrual cycle.

3. Incorporating Iron-Rich Foods:

Women are more prone to iron deficiency, especially during menstruation. Include iron-rich foods like lean meats, legumes, dark leafy greens, and fortified cereals to support energy levels and prevent anemia.

4. Calcium and Vitamin D Intake:

Women, particularly those in menopause or postmenopausal stages, need to pay attention to calcium and vitamin D intake for bone health. Incorporate dairy, fortified plant-based milk, and green leafy vegetables into the diet. Supplements or exposure to sunlight are two ways to get vitamin D.

5. Addressing Menopausal Changes:

Menopause can lead to changes in metabolism and an increased risk of insulin resistance. Consider incorporating more fiber-rich foods, lean proteins, and healthy fats to manage weight and hormonal fluctuations during this stage.

6. Mindful Eating Practices:
Women often face emotional and stress-related eating challenges. Encourage mindful eating practices to manage stress, emotional triggers, and prevent overeating. This may involve incorporating stress-reducing activities, such as meditation or yoga.

7. Customizing Caloric Intake:
Caloric needs vary based on age, activity level, and metabolic rate. Tailor the Blood Sugar Diet to individual calorie requirements, ensuring women are consuming enough energy to support their daily activities and metabolic demands.

8. Hydration:
Adequate hydration is crucial for women's health. Water intake can impact blood sugar

regulation and assist in weight management. Encourage regular water consumption throughout the day.

9. Consulting Healthcare Professionals:
Women with specific health conditions, such as polycystic ovary syndrome (PCOS) or gestational diabetes, may require further customization. Seeking advice from dietitians or medical specialists might offer tailored advice.

Hormonal Influences on Blood Sugar

Women's hormonal influences play a significant role in regulating blood sugar levels. Hormones such as estrogen and progesterone, which fluctuate throughout the menstrual cycle and other life stages, can impact insulin sensitivity and glucose metabolism. Here's an overview of how hormonal changes in women can influence blood sugar:

1. Menstrual Cycle:

Menstrual Phase (Days 1-5): During the menstrual phase, estrogen and progesterone levels are low. This can lead to increased insulin sensitivity, potentially making women more responsive to carbohydrates. It's essential to maintain a balanced diet and manage cravings during this phase.

Follicular Phase (Days 6-14): Estrogen begins to rise, leading to improved insulin sensitivity. Women may experience increased energy levels and better glucose tolerance during this phase.

Ovulatory Phase (Days 15-17): Estrogen peaks, and insulin sensitivity remains high. This phase may also coincide with increased energy and improved carbohydrate metabolism.

Luteal Phase (Days 18-28): Both estrogen and progesterone are elevated during the luteal phase. Insulin sensitivity may decrease, and some women may experience cravings for carbohydrates. Emphasizing complex carbohydrates, fiber, and nutrient-dense foods can help manage blood sugar levels.

2. Pregnancy:

During pregnancy, hormonal changes are significant. Insulin resistance naturally increases to provide the developing fetus with sufficient glucose. Women may experience gestational diabetes due to the increased demand for insulin. Monitoring blood sugar levels and adhering to a balanced diet is crucial during pregnancy to prevent complications.

3. Postmenopausal Changes:

After menopause, estrogen levels decline, leading to changes in metabolism and fat distribution. Insulin resistance may increase, raising the risk of Type 2 diabetes. It becomes crucial for women in postmenopausal stages to focus on maintaining a healthy weight, engaging in regular physical activity, and managing carbohydrate intake.

4. Polycystic Ovary Syndrome (PCOS):

PCOS is a hormonal disorder that can affect insulin sensitivity. Women with PCOS may have elevated levels of insulin, contributing to higher blood sugar levels. Lifestyle modifications, including a balanced diet and regular exercise, are essential in managing PCOS-related insulin resistance.

5. Hormone Replacement Therapy (HRT):

Women undergoing hormone replacement therapy, commonly used during menopause, may experience changes in insulin sensitivity. It's important to monitor blood sugar levels and adapt dietary habits accordingly.

6. Stress Hormones:

Stress hormones, such as cortisol, can impact blood sugar regulation. Chronic stress can lead to insulin resistance and higher blood sugar levels. Managing stress through relaxation techniques, exercise, and proper sleep is crucial for overall hormonal balance.

7. Individual Variations:

Each woman's response to hormonal fluctuations is unique. Some may be more sensitive to changes in insulin levels, while others may have more stable blood sugar throughout their menstrual cycle. Monitoring blood sugar levels and adjusting dietary choices based on individual responses is key.

Understanding and adapting to these hormonal influences on blood sugar can empower women to make informed choices about their diet and lifestyle. Regular monitoring, maintaining a balanced and nutrient-dense diet, and seeking guidance from healthcare professionals are essential components of managing blood sugar levels throughout different stages of a woman's life.

Special Considerations for Pregnant Women

Pregnancy is a time when blood sugar control becomes crucial for the health of both the mother and the developing baby. Here are special considerations and advice for pregnant women in blood sugar control:

1. Regular Monitoring:

Regularly monitor blood sugar levels as directed by healthcare providers. This helps in adjusting diet and medication as needed to maintain optimal blood sugar levels throughout pregnancy.

2. Balanced Diet:

A well-balanced diet consisting of a range of nutrient-dense foods should be your main priority. Make sure you're getting enough fats, proteins, and carbohydrates.

Choose complex carbohydrates with a low glycemic index (GI) to help manage blood sugar levels. Examples include whole grains, legumes, and vegetables.

3. Meal Timing and Frequency:

Throughout the day, have smaller, more frequent meals to help balance your blood sugar levels.

Avoid skipping meals, as this can lead to blood sugar fluctuations.

4. Limit Sugary Foods and Beverages:

Minimize the consumption of sugary foods and beverages. Opt for healthier snacks and drinks to avoid spikes in blood sugar levels.

5. Protein Intake:

Include adequate protein in each meal, as it helps stabilize blood sugar levels and supports the baby's growth.

6. Fiber-Rich Foods:

Choose fiber-rich foods, such as fruits, vegetables, and whole grains, to aid digestion and help regulate blood sugar.

7. Hydration:

Drink plenty of water throughout the day to be well-hydrated. Dehydration can affect blood sugar levels.

8. Regular Exercise:

Engage in moderate and safe exercise as recommended by healthcare providers. Regular physical activity can help regulate blood sugar levels and improve overall well-being.

9. Gestational Diabetes Testing:

Women at risk for gestational diabetes should undergo screening as recommended by healthcare providers. If diagnosed with gestational diabetes, careful monitoring and management become even more critical.

10. Medication Management:

If prescribed medication for gestational diabetes or other pre-existing conditions, follow the healthcare provider's instructions meticulously.

Insulin or oral medications may be necessary to control blood sugar levels, and adjustments may be needed as the pregnancy progresses.

11. Consult with Healthcare Providers:

Regularly consult with healthcare providers, including obstetricians, endocrinologists, and dietitians, to receive personalized guidance and support.

12. Weight Management:

Aim for healthy weight gain during pregnancy, as excessive weight gain can contribute to insulin resistance. Healthcare providers can provide individualized recommendations based on pre-pregnancy weight and health status.

13. Postpartum Monitoring:

Continue monitoring blood sugar levels after giving birth, as gestational diabetes increases the risk of developing Type 2 diabetes later in life.

14. Breastfeeding Benefits:

If possible, consider breastfeeding, as it may help with blood sugar control and offers numerous health benefits for both mother and baby.

Pregnant women should work closely with their healthcare team to develop a personalized plan for blood sugar control during pregnancy. Each woman's situation is unique, and individualized care is essential to ensure a healthy pregnancy and the well-being of both the mother and the baby.

Menopause and Blood Sugar

Menopause is a natural biological process marking the end of a woman's reproductive years, typically occurring in the late 40s or early 50s. During menopause, hormonal changes, specifically a decline in estrogen levels, can have implications for blood sugar regulation. Here are some insights into the relationship between menopause and blood sugar:

1. Insulin Sensitivity and Resistance:

Estrogen plays a role in maintaining insulin sensitivity. As estrogen levels decline during menopause, some women may experience a decrease in insulin sensitivity, potentially leading to insulin resistance.

Insulin resistance can result in higher blood sugar levels, increasing the risk of developing Type 2 diabetes.

2. Changes in Fat Distribution:

Menopause is associated with changes in body composition, including a tendency for increased abdominal fat. Abdominal fat is linked to insulin resistance and may contribute to elevated blood sugar levels.

3. Metabolic Rate and Weight Management:

Metabolic rate often decreases with age, and this, combined with hormonal changes, can make it more challenging to manage weight during and after menopause.

Maintaining a healthy weight through a balanced diet and regular exercise is crucial for blood sugar control.

4. Risk of Type 2 Diabetes:

The postmenopausal period is associated with an increased risk of developing Type 2 diabetes. Women should be vigilant about lifestyle factors, including diet and exercise, to mitigate this risk.

5. Importance of Regular Exercise:

Regular physical activity becomes even more critical during and after menopause. Exercise helps improve insulin sensitivity, manage weight, and reduce the risk of developing Type 2 diabetes.

6. Dietary Considerations:

Focus on a nutrient-dense, well-balanced diet that includes whole grains, lean proteins, healthy fats, and a variety of fruits and vegetables.

Monitor carbohydrate intake, choosing complex carbohydrates with a low glycemic index to help manage blood sugar levels.

7. Calcium and Vitamin D Intake:

Reduced estrogen levels can impact bone health. It's essential to ensure an adequate intake of calcium and vitamin D, either through diet or supplements, to support bone health.

8. Regular Blood Sugar Monitoring:

Women in menopause or postmenopause should monitor their blood sugar levels regularly, especially if they have other risk factors for Type 2 diabetes.

9. Hormone Replacement Therapy (HRT):

Some women opt for hormone replacement therapy to manage symptoms of menopause. HRT's impact on blood sugar can vary, and it's crucial to discuss potential effects with healthcare providers.

10. Stress Management:

Chronic stress can contribute to insulin resistance. Incorporate stress management techniques, such as mindfulness, meditation, or yoga, into daily life.

11. Regular Health Check-ups:

Regular check-ups with healthcare providers should include discussions about blood sugar control and overall metabolic health. This allows for early detection and intervention if any issues arise.

12. Personalized Approach:

Each woman's experience with menopause is unique. It's essential to tailor lifestyle modifications to individual needs, taking into account factors such as genetics, overall health, and personal preferences.

13. Educational Support:

Seek educational resources and support groups that focus on managing health during menopause. Staying informed and connected with others going through similar experiences can be beneficial.

Women navigating menopause should approach blood sugar control holistically, considering lifestyle factors such as diet, exercise, stress management, and regular monitoring. Working closely with healthcare providers ensures a personalized approach to maintain optimal metabolic health during and after menopause.

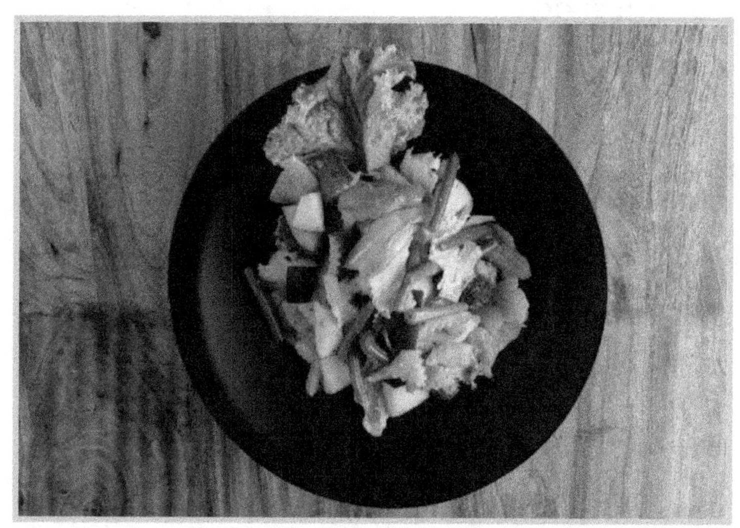

CHAPTER NINE

Creating your 14-Day Meal Plan

Building a Balanced Plate

Building a balanced plate is crucial for blood sugar control in women, as it helps regulate insulin levels and promotes overall health. Here are some general guidelines for creating a balanced plate:

Include Lean Proteins:
Pick lean protein sources including fish, chicken, tofu, lentils, and low-fat dairy products.
Protein encourages satiety and helps control blood sugar levels, which helps people avoid overindulging.

Incorporate Whole Grains:

Choose whole grains such as whole wheat, quinoa, brown rice, and oats.

Whole grains have a lower glycemic index, which means they cause a slower rise in blood sugar compared to refined grains.

Add Colorful Vegetables:

Include a variety of colorful, non-starchy vegetables in your meals.

Vegetables are rich in fiber, vitamins, and minerals, and they have a minimal impact on blood sugar levels.

Choose Healthy Fats:

Incorporate foods like avocados, almonds, seeds, and olive oil that are good sources of fat.

Healthy fats can help slow down the absorption of carbohydrates, preventing rapid spikes in blood sugar.

Watch Portion Sizes:

Pay attention to portion proportions to prevent overindulging.

Stable blood sugar levels can be achieved with eating smaller, more balanced meals throughout the day.

Limit Added Sugars:

Reduce the amount of added-sugar foods and beverages you consume.

Choose natural sources of sweetness like fruits when you have a sweet craving.

Include Fiber-Rich Foods:

Eat a lot of fruits, vegetables, whole grains, and legumes as well as other high-fiber foods.

In order to minimize sharp rises in blood sugar, fiber helps slow down the digestion and absorption of carbs.

Stay Hydrated:

Drink plenty of water throughout the day.

Water can help regulate hunger and is necessary for good health in general.

Consider the Glycemic Index:
Be aware of the glycemic index of foods.In general, foods having a lower glycemic index are better at controlling blood sugar.

Regular Meal Timing:
Aim for regular and consistent meal times.
This can help regulate blood sugar levels and prevent extreme fluctuations.

It's essential for individuals, including women, to work with their healthcare providers and registered dietitians to create a personalized and sustainable eating plan that meets their specific needs and health goals. Additionally, regular physical activity plays a crucial role in blood sugar management, so incorporating exercise into your routine is beneficial as well.

Meal Timing and Frequency

Meal timing and frequency play a significant role in blood sugar control. The goal is to maintain stable blood sugar levels throughout the day, which can be achieved by paying attention to when and how often you eat. Here are some considerations for meal timing and frequency to help regulate blood sugar:

Regular Meal Schedule:
Aim for a consistent meal schedule by eating meals and snacks at roughly the same times each day.
Regularity in eating helps the body anticipate and manage insulin release more effectively.

Balanced Meals:
Every meal should contain a mix of complex carbohydrates, healthy fats, and protein.
This balance helps slow down the absorption of sugars into the bloodstream, preventing rapid spikes in blood sugar.

Avoid Skipping Meals:

Skipping meals can lead to irregular blood sugar levels and increased likelihood of overeating later.

Eating regularly helps maintain energy levels and prevents extreme fluctuations in blood sugar.

Choose Nutrient-Dense Snacks:

If you need snacks between meals, opt for nutrient-dense options like fruits, vegetables, nuts, or yogurt.

Nutrient-dense snacks provide sustained energy without causing sharp increases in blood sugar.

Post-Exercise Nutrition:

Consider the timing of meals concerning physical activity.

Consuming a balanced meal or snack after exercise can help replenish glycogen stores and stabilize blood sugar levels.

Limit Late-Night Eating:

Aim to avoid eating large or high-carb meals right before bed.

Late-night eating can disrupt overnight blood sugar levels and impact sleep quality.

Grazing vs. Three Meals:

Some people find success with three balanced meals a day, while others prefer smaller, more frequent meals (grazing).

Experiment to find what works best for you, keeping in mind the importance of balance and moderation.

Listen to Hunger and Fullness Cues:

Observe the cues your body gives you about hunger and fullness.

Eating in response to physical hunger and stopping when satisfied can help regulate blood sugar and prevent overeating.

Consider Intermittent Fasting:

Some individuals may benefit from intermittent fasting, which involves cycles of eating and fasting.

Consult with a healthcare professional before adopting intermittent fasting, especially if you have existing health conditions.

Monitor Blood Sugar Levels:

Regularly monitor your blood sugar levels, especially if you have diabetes or other metabolic conditions.

Monitoring can provide valuable insights into how different foods and meal timings affect your blood sugar.

It's important to note that individual responses to meal timing and frequency can vary. Consulting with a healthcare professional or a registered dietitian can help tailor recommendations to your specific needs and health goals, particularly if you have conditions like diabetes.

Sample Meal Plans for Breakfast, Lunch, Dinner, and Snacks

Creating a sample meal plan for blood sugar control requires a personalized approach based on factors like individual preferences, dietary restrictions, and calorie needs. However, here's a general 14-day sample meal plan to provide you with some ideas. Keep in mind that portion sizes may need to be adjusted based on individual requirements.

Day	Breakfast	Lunch	Dinner	Snacks
1	Greek yogurt with berries and a sprinkle of almonds	Quinoa salad with mixed vegetables and grilled chicken	Baked salmon with steamed asparagus and a small sweet potato	Carrot sticks with hummus

2	Oatmeal with sliced strawberries and a tablespoon of chia seeds	Turkey and avocado wrap with a side salad	Stir-fried tofu with broccoli, bell peppers, and brown rice	Apple slices with a tablespoon of peanut butter
3	Scrambled eggs with spinach and whole grain toast	Lentil soup with a side of mixed greens	Grilled shrimp with quinoa and roasted zucchini	Plain popcorn

4	Smoothie with spinach, banana, and unsweetened almond milk	Grilled vegetable salad with feta cheese and a drizzle of balsamic vinaigrette	Baked chicken breast with steamed green beans and a small portion of wild rice	Mixed nuts
5	Whole grain toast with mashed avocado and a poached egg	Chickpea salad with cucumbers, tomatoes, and a lemon-tahini dressing	Turkey meatballs with zucchini noodles and marinara sauce	Edamame

| 6 | Cottage cheese with sliced peaches and a sprinkle of sunflower seeds | Quinoa and black bean stuffed bell peppers | Grilled salmon with sautéed spinach and a small sweet potato | Sugar snap peas with hummus |
| 7 | Chia seed pudding with unsweetened coconut and berries | Tuna salad lettuce wraps with a side of carrot and celery sticks | Baked tofu with roasted Brussels sprouts and quinoa | Plain yogurt with a drizzle of honey |

| 8 | Whole grain waffle with Greek yogurt and mixed berries | Spinach and feta omelet with a side of mixed greens | Grilled chicken skewers with bell peppers and onions, served with a small portion of brown rice | Sliced bell peppers with guacamole |
| 9 | Scrambled eggs with spinach and whole grain toast | Turkey and avocado wrap with a side salad | Baked salmon with steamed asparagus and a small sweet potato | Carrot sticks with hummus |

| 10 | Oatmeal with sliced strawberries and a tablespoon of chia seeds | Stir-fried tofu with broccoli, bell peppers, and brown rice | Lentil soup with a side of mixed greens | Apple slices with a tablespoon of peanut butter |
| 11 | Smoothie with spinach, banana, and unsweetened almond milk | Grilled vegetable salad with feta cheese and a drizzle of balsamic vinaigrette | Baked chicken breast with steamed green beans and a small portion of wild rice | Mixed nuts |

12	Whole grain toast with mashed avocado and a poached egg	Turkey meatballs with zucchini noodles and marinara sauce	Grilled salmon with sautéed spinach and a small sweet potato	Edamame
13	Cottage cheese with sliced peaches and a sprinkle of sunflower seeds	Baked tofu with roasted Brussels sprouts and quinoa	Tuna salad lettuce wraps with a side of carrot and celery sticks	Sugar snap peas with hummus

| 14 | Chia seed pudding with unsweetened coconut and berries | Whole grain waffle with Greek yogurt and mixed berries | Grilled chicken skewers with bell peppers and onions, served with a small portion of brown rice | Plain yogurt with a drizzle of honey |

These meal plans are designed to help manage blood sugar levels and provide a variety of nutritious and balanced meals. It's important for individuals to work with a doctor or a registered dietitian to create a meal plan that suits their specific needs. The Diabetes Plate Method can be used to create perfectly portioned meals with a healthy balance of vegetables, protein, and carbohydrates—without any counting, calculating, weighing, or measuring

CHAPTER TEN

Smart Grocery Shopping for Blood Sugar Management

Smart grocery shopping is crucial for effective blood sugar management, especially for individuals with diabetes or those aiming to maintain stable blood sugar levels. Here are some important things to think about:

Reading Food Labels

Carbohydrate Content: Focus on the total carbohydrate content per serving, as carbohydrates have the most significant impact on blood sugar levels. Look for foods with lower glycemic index (GI) values.

Fiber: Choose foods high in fiber, as it helps slow down the absorption of sugar and can contribute to better blood sugar control. Aim for whole grains, fruits, vegetables, and legumes.

Added Sugars: Be wary of added sugars, as they can quickly raise blood sugar levels. Check the ingredient list for terms like sucrose, high-fructose corn syrup, and other sweeteners.

Choosing the Right Ingredients

Entire Foods: Choose unprocessed, entire foods including fruits, vegetables, whole grains, and lean meats. These foods generally have a lower impact on blood sugar levels and provide essential nutrients.

Lean Proteins: Include lean proteins like poultry, fish, tofu, and legumes, as they can help stabilize blood sugar levels and promote satiety.

Good Fats: Include good fats from nuts, seeds, avocados, and olive oil, among other sources. These fats can slow down the digestion of carbohydrates, preventing rapid spikes in blood sugar.

Meal Preparation Tips

Portion Control: Be mindful of portion sizes to avoid overeating, as excessive intake of any food can impact blood sugar levels. Use measuring tools to help control portions.

Meal Planning: A balanced and nutrient-dense diet can be achieved by arranging your meals in advance. This can help you make healthier choices and avoid last-minute, less healthy options.

Cooking Methods: Choose cooking methods that don't add excessive fats or sugars.Low-oil methods like baking, sautéing, grilling, and steaming are excellent choices.

Snacking Smart: Have healthy snacks on hand, such as nuts, seeds, Greek yogurt, or cut vegetables. This can help stabilize blood sugar levels between meals.

Remember, it's essential to consult with a healthcare professional or a registered dietitian to create a personalized plan that suits your specific dietary needs and health goals.

Regular monitoring of blood sugar levels is also crucial to understand how different foods affect your body and to make adjustments accordingly.

CHAPTER ELEVEN

Recipes for Blood Sugar Control

Managing blood sugar levels is important for overall health, especially for women. Here are some recipes for each meal that focus on balanced nutrition and can help in managing blood sugar levels:

Breakfast Option

1. Greek Yogurt Parfait:

Ingredients:

1 cup Greek yogurt (unsweetened)

1/2 cup fresh berries (blueberries, strawberries)

1 tablespoon chia seeds

1/4 cup chopped nuts (almonds, walnuts)

1 teaspoon honey (optional)

Instructions:

In a bowl or glass, layer Greek yogurt, berries, chia seeds, and nuts.

Drizzle honey on top if desired.

2. Vegetable Omelette:

Ingredients:

2 eggs

1/4 cup diced bell peppers

1/4 cup diced tomatoes

1/4 cup chopped spinach

Salt and pepper to taste

Instructions:

In a bowl, whisk together eggs, salt, and
pepper.

Pour the egg mixture into a pan over medium
heat.

Add vegetables and cook until the eggs are
set.

Lunch Options

1. Quinoa Salad:

Ingredients:

1 cup cooked quinoa

1/2 cup cherry tomatoes, halved

1/4 cup cucumber, diced

1/4 cup feta cheese

2 tablespoons olive oil

Lemon juice, salt, and pepper to taste

Instructions:

In a bowl, combine quinoa, cherry tomatoes, cucumber, and feta cheese.

Drizzle with olive oil and lemon juice. Season with salt and pepper.

2. Grilled Chicken and Vegetable Skewers:

Ingredients:

Chicken breast, cut into chunks

Bell peppers, zucchini, cherry tomatoes

Olive oil, garlic, salt, and pepper

Instructions:

Thread chicken and vegetables onto skewers.

Mix olive oil, minced garlic, salt, and pepper. Brush over skewers.

Grill until chicken is cooked through and vegetables are tender.

Dinner Options

1. Baked Salmon with Asparagus:

Ingredients:

Salmon fillets

Asparagus spears

Lemon, garlic, salt, and pepper

Instructions:

Place salmon and asparagus on a baking sheet.

Drizzle with olive oil, squeeze lemon juice, and season with garlic, salt, and pepper.

Bake until salmon flakes easily.

2. Cauliflower Rice Stir-Fry:

Ingredients:

Cauliflower rice

Mixed vegetables (broccoli, carrots, peas)

Tofu or lean protein

Low-sodium soy sauce

Instructions:

Stir-fry cauliflower rice, mixed vegetables, and tofu or protein.

Add low-sodium soy sauce for flavor.

Snack Options

1. Hummus with Veggie Sticks:

Ingredients:

Carrot sticks, cucumber slices, bell pepper strips

Hummus

Instructions:

Dip vegetable sticks into hummus for a satisfying snack.

2. Cottage Cheese with Berries:

Ingredients:

Cottage cheese

Mixed berries (strawberries, blueberries)

Instructions:

Top cottage cheese with mixed berries for a protein-packed snack.

Smoothies Option

1. Green Smoothie:

Ingredients:

Spinach or kale

Banana

Greek yogurt

Almond milk

Chia seeds

Instructions:

Blend spinach, banana, Greek yogurt, almond milk, and chia seeds until smooth.

2. Berry Protein Smoothie:

Ingredients:

Mixed berries (strawberries, raspberries, blueberries)

Protein powder

Almond milk

Instructions:

Blend mixed berries, protein powder, and almond milk for a delicious protein smoothie.

Remember to consult with a healthcare professional or a nutritionist for personalized advice based on individual health conditions.

CONCLUSION

IThe Blood Sugar Diet Solution for Women presents a compelling and empowering approach to managing blood sugar levels, promoting overall health, and addressing the unique needs of women. Through a combination of insightful nutritional guidance, practical lifestyle tips, and a deep understanding of the female body, this book provides a comprehensive solution for women looking to take control of their blood sugar and achieve lasting well-being. As readers embark on this transformative journey, they are not only equipped with valuable knowledge but also inspired to make sustainable changes that will positively impact their health and vitality. With a focus on balance, nourishment, and mindful living, this book serves as a beacon of empowerment, guiding women towards a healthier and more vibrant life.

Crucially, the concluding chapters emphasize the importance of long-term commitment and mindful living. Rather than offering a quick fix, the book advocates for a lasting transformation rooted in self-care. Readers are left with a profound appreciation for the interconnectedness of their dietary choices, blood sugar levels, and overall vitality. Ultimately, "The Blood Sugar Diet Solution for Women" concludes as more than a guide – it stands as a beacon of empowerment, steering women toward a healthier and more balanced life through an intelligent and sustainable approach to managing their blood sugar